# YOUR PILLS WON'T SAVE YOU!

## THE POWER TO REVERSE DISEASE

*Your Roadmap to Transformational Healing*

DR. MINNI MALHOTRA

M.D., ABFM, ABAARM, IFMCP

DR. MINNI MALHOTRA
M.D., ABFM, ABAARM, IFMCP

Published By

Cronus Media Ventures, LLC and Epoch Publishing

ISBN: 978-0-9963197-9-9

Printed in the United States of America
First Printing 2020
First Edition 2020

10 9 8 7 6 5 4 3 2 1

# YOUR PILLS WON'T SAVE YOU!

THE POWER TO REVERSE DISEASE

# Disclaimer

This book is designed to provide general education and guidelines and, is not intended to represent personalized medical advice or specific recommendations. The information presented here is not intended to replace professional medical advice, diagnosis or treatment.

Readers with specific questions regarding a medical condition should always consult a registered physician or other qualified health professional. Even if this book covers one or more of the issues you are experiencing, always seek medical advice and do not delay medical treatment.

Please call 911 or call your doctor immediately if you are experiencing a medical emergency.

Direct any questions to Dr. Minni Malhotra and Anchor Wellness Center at info@anchorwellnesscenter.com

# TESTIMONIALS

*My major issue was hormonal imbalance, mainly the thyroid from a recent blood test. I was feeling drowsy in the mornings, mid afternoon crash, trouble loosing weight, brain fog, etc. But it's never one thing, the body is intricately interwoven, there's always a culmination of a multitude of imbalances. Immediately I began the elimination program, and started to feel better. Then came the Detox stage, and a week into that, my energy started to sore. I knew I was on the right tract. Dr. Minni is very knowledgeable, she not only relies on blood test, but a multitude of whole body results before making a proper diagnosis and treatment program. A normal MD has about 15 minutes per patient. How can you properly treat anything? With Dr. Minni, she spends hours reviewing results, researching, and properly treating with the culmination of multitudes of test. Her staff is personable and efficient. I would highly recommend Anchor Wellness who truly wants to obtain maximum health, not just cover up symptoms with a "band aid" like approach in which a lifetime of drugs is the prescription. People do not have high blood pressure, diabetes, nor high cholesterol because their bodies lack drugs. I choose nutrition and exercise in order to maintain a lifestyle without a lifetime sentence of drugs!*

---

***N.I.***

*I have Hashimoto's Disease, so losing weight has always been an issue for me. So far I've lost over 20lbs, and I've gained a ton of energy. Dr Minni and her staff are very knowledgeable and willing to answer any questions you may have. They are there to help you every step of the way. I have been given more information about my specific health concerns from Dr Minni and her staff than I've ever been given from any medical doctor before. The program is easy to understand and follow. Classes are held regularly to help you understand how nutrition works and proper exercise techniques. This program is worth every penny and more.*

---

***N.L. W.***

*So, for us, this is a lifestyle change. This is about not being sick and old, like our parents. Both of my parents have been diagnosed with Alzheimer's, and we're not gonna be sick and old. We have to get old, but we don't have to be sick, and that's why we're here. That, and making our hormones balance, which is good. Wonderful.*

*So, thank you for showing us how to change what we have been brought up to believe, and the things that we were taught wrong, that we're having to totally, totally, learn a whole new way of eating.*

---

***M.L.B.***

*I joined the program because I finally decided to make the decision that I was sick and tired of being sick and tired. I focus so much on what I look like physically that I just get depression. I went into these vicious cycles of hard-core dieting and binging. It wasn't healthy. I decided I need to fix the inside of me. So I took half of me in good. I'm not the smallest I've ever been, but I'm the happiest I've ever been and have the most energy I thought I ever could have. So I'm very happy with this program. Thank you so much.*

---

**M.**

*I wanted to go on path of more healthy living and holistic healing and wellness, so this was the perfect path, I found.*

*I was 30 pounds overweight, and now I've lost that weight, so I'm on a projectory that is positive and it's very helpful. I learned a lot.*

*My weight made me sluggish, it made me a unhappy. It made me uncomfortable, and I didn't have as much energy as I do now.*

*The program helped me learn what to eat or not to eat, how to shop at a grocery store. The program helped me learn the importance of hormones and hormone health, and the program helped me learn how your body can heal itself if you eat right and if you take care of yourself, get enough sleep, and you minimize your stress.*

*I find that I deal with my stress at work in healthier ways from this program, and professionally and personally, I feel more secure in pursuing my overall health goal to improve my health and to do more runs and races and stuff.*

---

**Y.O.**

*I'm Kim. Okay, both of my parents died of heart disease and both of my siblings died of cancer. That's really why I came because I don't want to have either one of those. I'm a cancer survivor myself. When I heard Dr. Minni, I thought I need to do whatever I can do to be the best I could be. Thank you Dr Minni for your help on putting me on this path.*

---

***K.***

*I'm 59 years old. I've been participating in the Anchor Wellness peak program for about a year. My health before that, I'll just tell you that I was pretty poor at maintaining my health for several years.*

*My blood pressure was very high and I also had low,... my blood tests came out with low testosterone. So, those two things were the things that were most trying. I had a vitamin deficiency as well. So these were my symptoms heading into the program ... high blood pressure, overweight, low testosterone, and low Vitamin D.*

*I lost about 50 pounds, and at the time before I entered the program I was feeling my age. I was feeling ... well, I'm 59 ... I kinda felt like I was 65.*

*I do enjoy better sleep at night. That's one of the benefits I have. I don't snore anymore.*

*I think the biggest thing is I do feel more fit. I guess the bad side of things, I had buy a new wardrobe.*

*My skin actually feels better. My circulation feels better. You can see purple veins and things in my skin before ... that they're not there anymore.*

*I play the violin. So, one of the other things I noticed too was when I play the violin, your violin has to be help up on your shoulder. It's much easier now and I think flexibility, loss of weight, higher energy level, better sleep and more alert.*

---

***Ivan***

*This has been a very significant thing for us, my wife and I. Not only losing weight was a big, I lost 40 pounds. I feel much more energetic than I have. I can't remember when I had this much energy and I'm out running my 30 something employees and climbing on rows and things that I haven't any done in a long time.*

*That's a very exciting thing, very exciting thing to be able to walk up the stairs without panting. It's a big deal for me....*

---

***M.B.***

*As a Christian I believe that God always guide us to what we need in life and I'm glad He guide me to Dr. Malhotra. I'm just happy that I did it, because I feel much, much, much better. I'm happy because my life has changed for the best.*

---

***N.S.***

*I am 85 years old, I tell you I as slowly dying when I went for her seminar. I just couldn't get up, I was nervous, I could hardly walk, I could nothing, I was just slowly dying.. But now I have come back alive!! I really thank Dr Minni for giving me my life back*

---

***Ruth***

*I have previously tried every diet in the books. Tops, weight watchers, liquid diet for a year. I even had my stomach stapled. At Anchor Wellness Center I have learned what my body needs to stay healthy. When I started the program, I couldn't take the one flight of stairs, had to stop and catch my breath. Now I am taking stairs 12 times in 30 minutes for my exercise, almost running up. In about 4 months I have lost about 30 pounds.*

---

***S.S.***

*My name is C.H. I had just lost my husband a few months ago and I did not want to become a couch potato. I wanted to live a life, do things. I saw her on FaceBook and she drew me in. When I listened to her speech, it was as if she was speaking to me. I thought this what I want to do. She has helped me more than anyone else. I love how I feel she has gotten me to a place I di =d not know existed. It has been great....*

---

***C.H.***

*When I came to Dr. Malhotra, I was very very sick. I had been on medical leave for many months and was about to lose my job. My fatigue was severe, I had endometriosis, chronic Lyme disease, Celiac disease and I had auto-immune rash all over my body, spots on my chest and on my back. I have been on the program for 4 months now. I have been able to go back to work. I am getting stronger all the time and I have improved my life. I have colleagues, who have health issues of their own, coming to me asking for help because they can see the difference and notice the change in my life.*

---

**S.B.**

# TABLE OF CONTENTS

# Preface

When Sharry Bowman (name changed), age 40 years, came to see me in July 2016, she had already been on medical leave for several months. Trying more than 21 Antibiotics, Anti-Depressants, Anti-Anxiety drugs and multiple supplements over last 2 years, she was not getting any better. With expenses piling up, she was on the verge of losing her job, her house, and a personal sense of freedom. A triple jeopardy defined.

We took her detailed history, asking very specific questions about her diet, lifestyle, early childhood illnesses, stresses, and recent health challenges. She suffered from severe fatigue, chronic Lyme disease, Celiac disease, Endometriosis, plus she had an autoimmune condition leading to rashes and or spots all over her body.

As is typical of our approach, we ran a battery of specific functional medicine tests, concurrently putting her on a structured Elimination diet. Her test results showed a variety of underlying gut problems, allergies and sensitivities to many foods including gluten which were causing significant inflammatory response in her body. Once we started treating her for these problems using a holistic approach including prescribing nutrient supplements, she was soon on the road to recovery. Sharry is already a changed person: back to work, resumed her normal life and is looking forward to the future with a very positive and optimistic frame of mind.

This is but one of the many success stories that I have encountered in my Functional medicine practice. We are continuing to successfully address conditions such as Diabetes, Thyroid Disorders, Digestive Disorders (IBS, GERD, etc), Elevated Cholesterol, Autoimmune disease, ADD, ADHD, Cognitive decline, Adrenal Fatigue, Hormone Imbalance, Low Libido, Lupus and many more.

Before I took this fork in the road towards Functional Medicine, I had a thriving Family Medicine practice. However, events in my professional and private life made me rethink my whole approach to Health, Vitality and Aging. At a professional level, I worried that I was not able to truly resolve the underlying pathology of my patients. Sure, I was able to provide a band aid, a drug to address the symptoms of their disease, and then often more drugs to address the (side) effects of the first drug and so on and so forth.

At a personal level, I have genetic obesity in my family, and my husband has a family history of diabetes, high cholesterol, heart disease and hypertension. With my propensity for obesity and my husband's genetic risks, our children were also predisposed to gaining weight and associated chronic ailments. For instance, our daughter was diagnosed with Polycystic Ovarian Syndrome (PCOS) at the tender age of ten. Every Physician I consulted, wanted to prescribe her multiple medications. I, myself being in the business of prescribing medications, was very wary of potential side effects of these medications.

I started researching for alternate options to take a more holistic approach towards patient care and effectively deal with the underlying causes of various chronic ailments, which is how I discovered Functional Medicine, and changed my whole perspective. I went back to school for rigorous training in various facets of Functional Medicine and started my own practice in this arena.

I can personally attest that this journey with my patients has been a very gratifying experience; it has changed their lives for the better, and really touched me to the core. People in their 20s, all the way to an 80-year-old lady who wanted her memory to be sharper and did not want to live with the aches and pains. She said, "if I die tomorrow, I want to die walking, talking, living and laughing." When she came to me, in her own words "I was slowly dying, but now I am back alive...". Today she is alive, full of energy and enthusiasm, and can't wait to get on with her day, everyday!

If it takes 15-20 years to develop a chronic disease, it's not going to go away by ingesting a few pills. You have to do something different. You have to get to the root cause and address that root cause. Human body is a very complex machine, and a whole array of factors - genetics, environment, mental, spiritual and physical health — all coming together to make a unique human experience for each one of us.

As you read this guide, ask yourself the following questions:

1. Does this make sense to me?
2. Am I ready to apply this approach to restore my health?

If the answer is yes, please give us a call and get on the path to Transformational Healing.

Sincerely,

Dr. Minni Malhotra, MD

Board Certified Family Practitioner

Anti-Aging Medicine Expert (ABAARM Certified)

Restorative Medicine Expert (ABAARM Certified)

Institute of Functional Medicine Certified Physician (IFMCP)

Email: drminni@anchorwellnesscenter.com

Phone: 832-246-8437

# Part I

*"Those who think they have no time for healthy eating will sooner or later have to find time for illness."*

# 1. We Have Healthcare Crisis Today

Here is a paradox. We have some of the best medical clinics, hospitals, fitness centers. We have high quality foods available at affordable costs – and, what's more - *we have lots of it.* However, while technically we advance medically, we grow sicker as a nation.

**Heart health:**

Horribly, someone has a *heart attack* every 34 seconds. And every 60 seconds, someone in the United States dies from a heart attack or stroke.

**Metabolic health:**

It is hard to believe, but 50 percent of us are now *prediabetic* or have full-blown diabetes.

**Immune health:**

A staggering one in two men and one in three women are projected to get *cancer* at some point in their life. Autoimmune *diseases* are now the third leading cause of death and disease in the world—affecting over 50 million Americans and millions more struggling with autoimmune-inflammation spectrum problems.

**Brain health:**

Nearly 20 percent of adult *suffer* from a diagnosable mental disorder. Depression is now the leading *cause* of disability worldwide. Anxiety disorders affect more than 40 million Americans and Alzheimer's disease is the sixth-leading *cause* of death in the United States. Autism and autism spectrum disorders (ASD) have *skyrocketed* over a short period of time; from an estimated one in 10,000 children in 1970 to one in 68 today representing a nearly 150 times increase.

# 2. We Have An Epidemic Of Chronic Illness

**The Reality**

These Diseases Don't Start "All of a sudden"

- ✓ Heart Disease has been shown to start in our youth (20-40 years before diagnosis).
- ✓ Cancer has been shown to start 15-30 years before diagnosis.
- ✓ Alzheimer's has been shown to start 30-50 years before diagnosis.
- ✓ Diabetes can start in the form of pre-diabetes 10-20 years years before diagnosis.

NOTE: Degenerative diseases have no medical "cure".

WORLD HEALTH DISEASE STATISTICS & TRENDS 2014

The Centers for Disease Control and Prevention estimates that one in two adults has at least one chronic condition such as heart disease, type 2 diabetes, hypertension, cancer, or arthritis. Chronic illness is now also linked to seven out of every 10 deaths in the United States.

A huge percentage of our population is taking medication that is ***primarily designed to mask symptoms instead of curing underlying issues.*** Did you know that the US spends more than $3.2 trillion per year on health care costs? When we look at the next 10 countries on the list, this is way more than what they spend – *combined.* And 75% of this cost is towards treating Chronic diseases.

Conditions like obesity, type 2 diabetes, and cancer are characterized by a series of complex, multilayered symptoms that take years to develop and can affect every biological system, including circulation, immunity, and hormonal and neurological health. By the time most people are diagnosed with a persistent condition, they need a full-scale intervention.

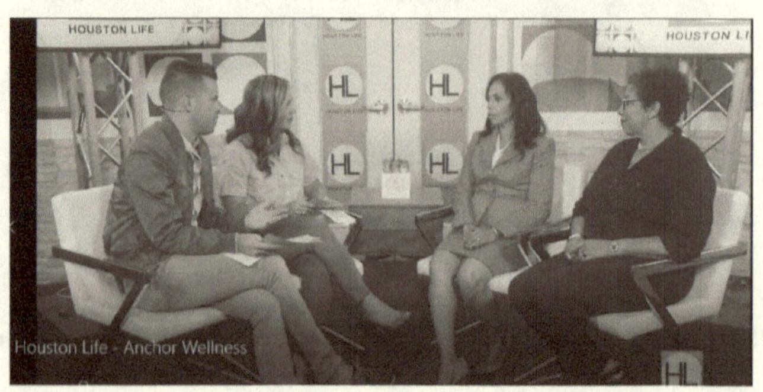

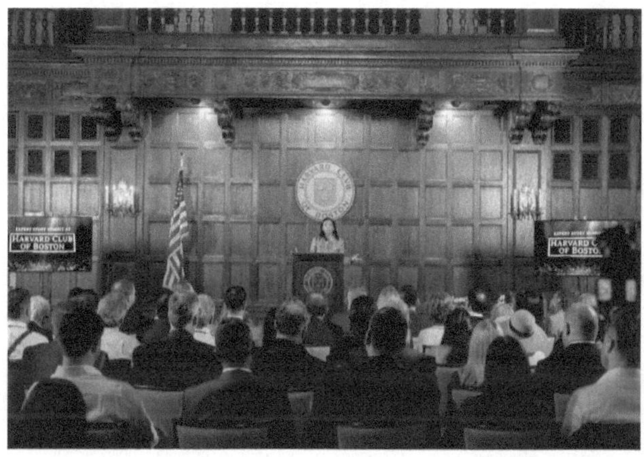


It is important to know what sort of person has a disease than to know what sort of disease a person has ---- Hippocrates

*"Just because you're not sick doesn't mean you're healthy."*

# 3. We Don't Have A Healthcare System, We Have A Disease Management System

Matching a drug to a disease is a big part of the typical physician's job. It works like this: You get sick. You go to the doctor. The doctor runs tests or recognizes your symptoms. You're given a prescription to take to the drugstore. Sometimes the drug works wonders. Often, it does not; particularly if you are dealing with is a chronic disease or condition. And quite often, the drug has side effects.

Practitioners in the hyper-specialized, overbooked world of conventional medicine, sometimes do not have the time or inclination to adopt the wider perspective of prevention and seeking proactive solutions.

A doctor of conventional medicine is essentially trained to give you a label for the disease, give the right ICD code and provide expensive prescription medication to treat its symptoms. There is little, if any, effort to restore our bodies to full health.

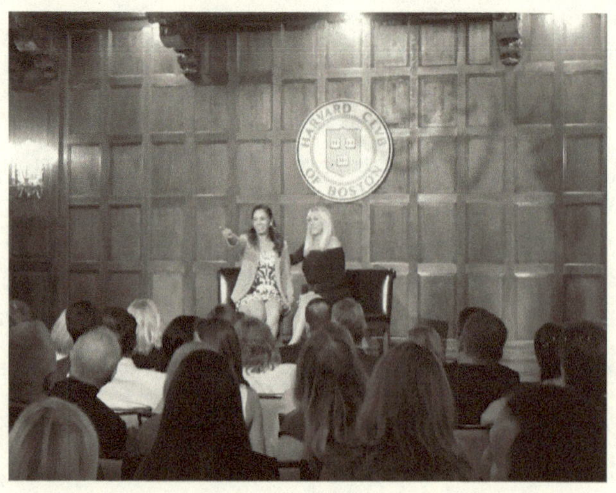


*"Let Food be Thy Medicine and Medicine be Thy Food."*

*– Hippocrates*

## 4. We Are What We Eat

We are constantly bombarded with advertisements for food that *looks* incredibly tasty but is made of some of the *worst* things we can put into our bodies. Equally true is that most of are prone to seeking "therapy" from day-to-day stresses by indulgence in junk food. We give into the temptations before us and gorge on junk food while expecting our bodies to continue functioning as normal.

Food is fuel for the body and mind. Our bodies are incredible machines, able to process a variety of foods in moderation but can also breakdown with constant barrage of unhealthy food choices. Once that happens, we go to our medical practitioners, waving our health insurance under the delusion of expecting a "cure" but more often than not, the physician is able to provide only symptomatic relief.

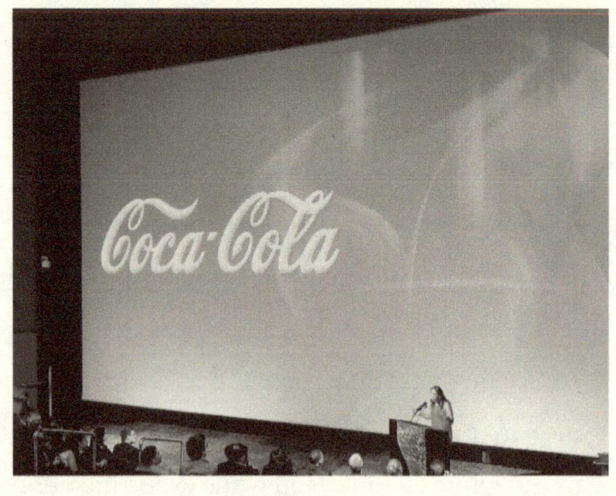


*"Healing is a matter of time, but it is sometimes also a matter of opportunity."*

*– Hippocrates*

# 5. How Traditional Medicine Is Falling Short

Conventional medicine is very good at acute care, be it pneumonia, a fractured limb, or a multitude of one-off conditions needing immediate treatment. Indeed, we have the some of the best Doctors and best facilities in the world to treat such ailments. However, using the same crisis care driven mentality for treating Chronic diseases leaves a lot to be desired. Conventional medicine can fall short in the early identification and long-term management of chronic illness, including the kinds of digestive, metabolic, hormonal, and cardiovascular disorders in which many functional-medicine doctors specialize.

Let's take a closer look at how traditional medicine might be failing you and your health and why you shoud consider investing in Wellness.

**1. Lack of personalization**

Your care is generally not custom-designed for you. You come in with symptoms, they are matched to the corresponding Code and a drug or a procedure corresponding to that Code. Each person on this earth is unique; genetics, biochemical make-up and epigenetics play a crucial role in eliciting these differences. What we need is personalized, precision medicine tailored specifically to you and your lifestyle.

**2. Addressing symptoms vs. the root cause of dysfunction**

Typically, your medications are only *managing* your symptoms, they are *not resolving* the underlying dysfunction in your body. A drug may initially make you feel better by masking the symptoms but non-resolution of the underlying cause of the symptoms will continue to put more and more stress on your body and worsen the condition. Finding out the underlying cause of your symptoms is critical to develop a personalized healthcare regime that works and is sustainable.

**3. (Side) Effects of Prescription medication.**

According to the *Journal of American Medical Association*, over 100,000 people die every year, simply by using their prescription medication *as directed.* Not from overdosing or taking the wrong drug, but from the side effects of the "right drug."

Typically, you take a medication to control a symptom. However, the drug has its own side effects, so you take a 2nd medication to manage the "side" effects of the first medication. For example, you may be on a medication that causes high blood pressure as one of its side-effects. This means you now have to take blood pressure medication too. And then have other symptoms "caused" by combination of these 2 drugs, and you are put on a third medication.

Let's look at the side effects of a very common anti-anxiety medication: clumsiness or unsteadiness, drowsiness, being forgetful, changes in patterns and rhythms of speech, irritability, loss of interest, feeling sad or empty, difficulty with coordination, trouble concentration, weakness and even suicide. And yes, there's also the increased risk of violent tendencies including harm to others. So, this drug – like many other drugs – messes with your brain.

Why would anyone want to suffer from these kinds of side effects *while* dealing with anxiety? Isn't it better to *treat* the anxiety instead of masking what's actually causing it?

Instead of letting pharmaceuticals rewire your brain and cause permanent damage, it is time for you to take your healthcare into your own hands for a more personalized, holistic approach and treat the causes of anxiety and address them.

*On a related note, chronic disease can often accentuate mental disorders, and a prolonged depressive state can lead to chronic ailments - a vicious cycle indeed!*

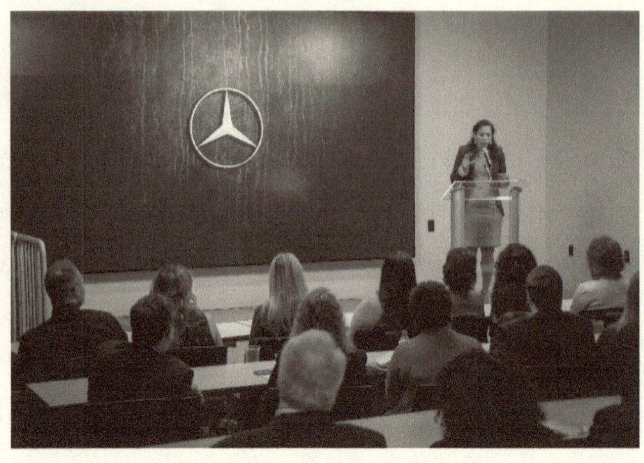

*"Take care of your body. It's the only place you have to live."*

*– Jim Rohn*

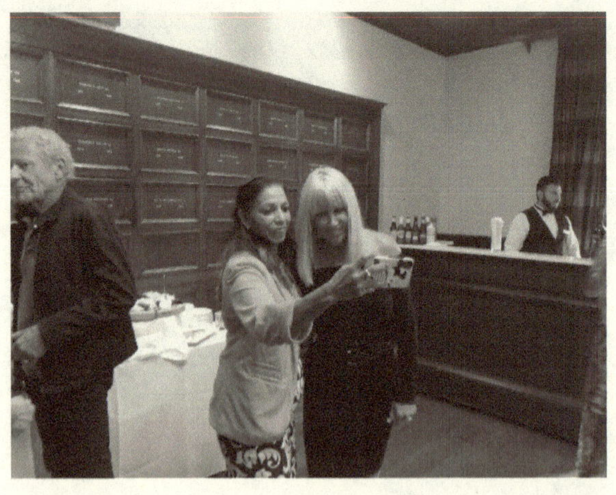

*He who has health has hope, and he who has hope has everything."*

*– Arabiab Proverrb*

# 6. Invest Now Or Pay Later

**Invest Now, Or Pay Later.**

**Disease Strips Performance & Drains The Bank**

- ✓ **Heart Disease costs $1,051,302,04 per person** (U.S. Preventative Service Task Force, 2007)
- ✓ **Cancer - New drugs cost over $100,000.00 per year with a $138,384.65 average expenditure** (ACS Cancer Fact and Figures 2012)
- ✓ **Alzheimer's costs $174,000.00 per person** (Alzheimer's Association, 2012)
- ✓ **Diabetes costs $13,700.00 per year, $174B in '07 to $245B in 2012 a 41% increase** (Diabetes.org 2013)

**US HEALTH DISEASE STATISTICS & TRENDS 2014**

In the United States, we spend almost 1 trillion dollars per year on direct medical costs to treat chronic ailments. At an individual level, the cost of treating such diseases through conventional care can quickly add-up. In extreme cases, such costs can drain hard-earned lifelong savings, and lead to bankruptcies.

Let's not forget the intangible costs:

*What is the cost of inability to spend time with your spouse, your children, your grandchildren or your loved ones because of sickness?*

*What is the cost of your inability to play Tag with your Grandchildren?*

*What is the cost of inability to be intimate with your spouse or significant other because of your illness?*

*What is the cost of inability to travel with your friends or family due to an infirmity?*

*And what is the cost of these people on the other end, who may not be sick but bear the unbearable cost of watching their loved one whither away?*

# 7. Perception vs Reality

There is a misconception that Functional Medicine is expensive. In fact, when you consider the long-term costs of chronic disease management - medications, co-pays, hospital stays, surgeries.., and all the intangible "costs" mentioned earlier - Functional Medicine is incredibly affordable.

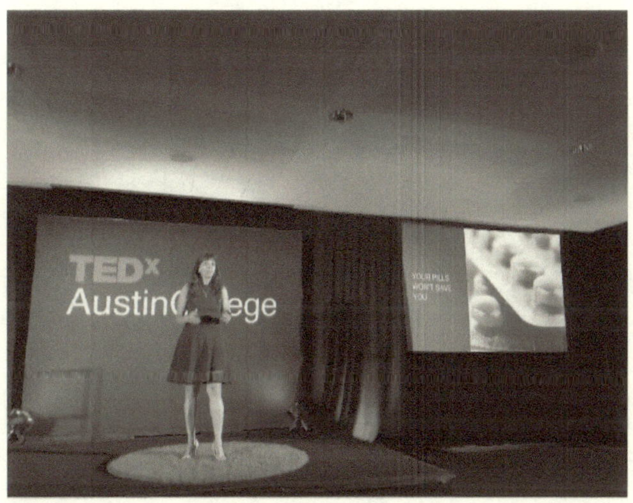

*Health is a state of body. Wellness is a state of being."*

*– J Stanford*

# PART II

*"You can't exercise your way out of bad diet."*

*– Dr Mark Hyman*

# 8. FUNCTIONAL MEDICINE - YOUR ROADMAP TO HEALTH AND VITALITY

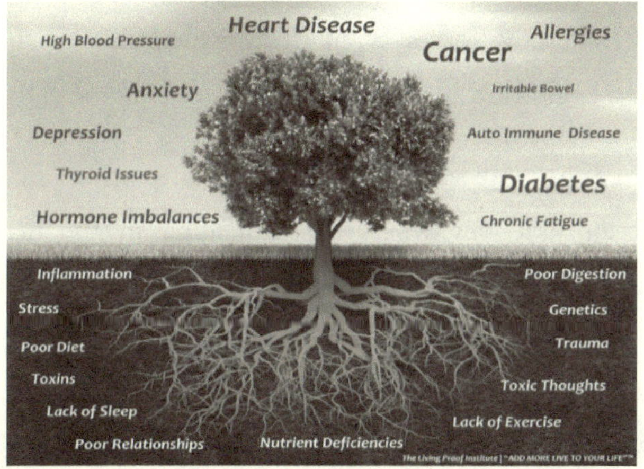


In Dr Hyman's own admission, when the head of the Cleveland Clinic approached functional medicine pioneer Mark Hyman, MD, several years ago about starting an institute devoted to functional medicine, Dr. Hyman actually tried to talk him out of it. "He said, 'Toby, you don't want me there. Because, if I go there I'm going to be disruptive. I'm going to tell you that most of what you are doing is based on an outdated paradigm of disease that in many cases creates more harm than good. I would want to implement programs that are going to empty out half your hospitals, clear out most of your procedure rooms, and reduce hospital stays and doctor visits dramatically". Toby Cosgrove, who oversaw the Cleveland Clinic from 2004 to 2017 and now serves as an executive advisor to the $8 billion healthcare system, was undaunted. He told Dr

Hyman he realized medicine was going in a different direction. He saw what was happening in the field of functional medicine and realized that's where the future was. In September of 2014, the Cleveland Clinic Center for Functional Medicine (CCCFM) opened, making the Cleveland Clinic the first mainstream institution to prominently incorporate the functional-medicine model.

As practitioners of Functional Medicine:

**We see the paradox in mainstream medicine.**

The United States spends more on health care than the next 10 top-spending countries combined! And

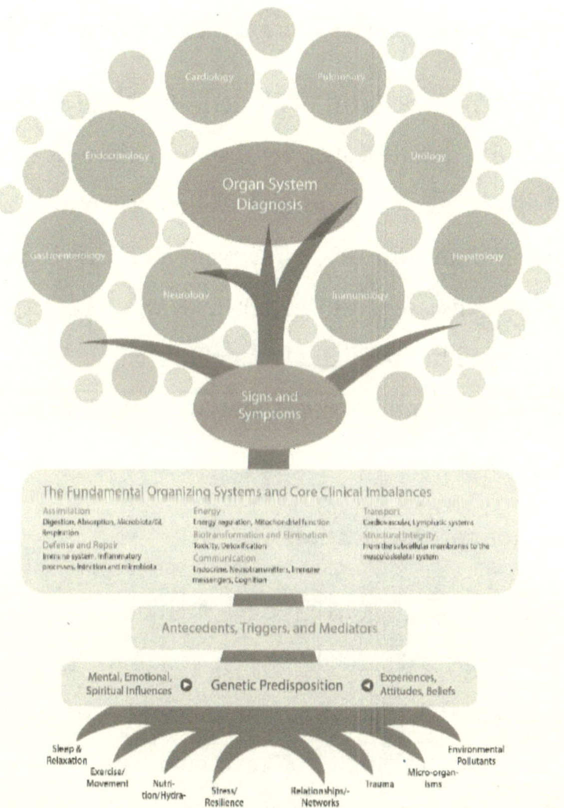


Personalizing Lifestyle and Environmental Factors

even though we spend trillions of dollars we rank last among all industrialized nations when it comes to living long, healthy lives.

**We realize no one is sick from a medication deficiency.**

A shocking 81 percent of Americans take at least one medication a day. But just because something is common, that does not mean it is normal. When it comes to chronic and autoimmune disease, mainstream medicine is trained to diagnose a disease and match it with a corresponding medication. This medicinal matching game leaves many frustrated when nothing changes with their health but a growing *prescription list.*

**We are not anti-medication**

We recognize that conventional medications have saved millions of lives especially when it comes to infectious diseases such as pneumonia, malaria and smallpox. Advancements in modern medicine have brought us lifesaving procedures, especially in emergency care. We just ask the question: What is our most effective option that causes the least amount of side effects? For some, a medication may fit this criterion. But a lot of the time, conventional pharmaceuticals are not the best choice.

**We realize our DNA is not our destiny.**

Research like the Danish Twin Study has shown that over 90 percent of our longevity is determined by the choices we make—not our genetics. Sure, people can have a genetic predisposition for certain diseases (most of us do) but those genes may not be expressed if they are not triggered by the epigenetic and lifestyle factors. In other words, pre-disposed does not necessarily translate into pre-destined.

**We believe the best medicine may be at the end of our forks.**

We strongly believe that diet has a major role to play in the prevention of onset, management and remission of various chronic diseases.

We work with our patients to develop dietary guidelines after extensive testing on their individual physiological profile.

Ten years from now,
make sure you
can say that
you chose your life,
you didn't settle for it.

# 9. Receive A Personalized Diagnosis

If you're reading this book, you may be searching for answers to one or more of the following questions:

- Why do I feel tired all the time?
- Am I supposed to feel so anxious?
- Why is my brain so foggy?
- Why can't I seem to lose weight even though I exercise?
- Will I always feel so sluggish?
- Do I need to take these medications lifelong?

In order to determine why you are feeling this way, it's important to go beyond the surface (without medication!) to find out exactly what's causing your symptoms.

Functional Medicine utilizes a wide array of cutting-edge diagnostic testing to help us see the bigger picture. When a traditional physician runs standard blood work, they are looking for an already established disease process. Generally, action is taken only when the lab results are out of the normal range. The trouble with this is that many people might not have an actual disease yet, but they are already suffering from some of the chronic symptoms and they are trending towards it.

Why wait until damage has been done? Functional medicine lab testing aims to prevent disease before it happens by assessing patterns of imbalance which, without intervention, will end up yielding chronic disease.

These are some of the tests that we routinely use to evaluate our patients.

- **Genetic Profile_**– This helps to understand your genetic makeup and customize the wellness plan to you individually.
- **Comprehensive Stool Analysis** - The test looks for markers of inflammation and malabsorption making it an essential test for those with inflammatory bowel disease, cardiovascular disease, diabetes, autoimmune issues and weight problems. This test also reveals the health of the gut's ecology (good and bad bacteria levels). The analysis detects

yeast, parasites, and toxins that cause antibiotic-associated diarrhea.

- **Small Dense LDL Particles** - In the simplistic view of traditional medicine, LDL is simply the bad Cholesterol. LDL particles carry cholesterol to different parts of the body and they can be large and fluffy or small and dense. The small LDL particles are more accurate predictors of heart health. The denser your particles are, the more damage they can cause, and can increase your risk for stroke and heart attack.
- **Telomere Length** - Telomeres are at the end of chromosomes and help encourage healthy cell function. As you get older, telomeres shorten and can cause chronic disease. By examining the length of telomeres, we can see how quickly your body is aging, and develop solutions to potentially slow-down the accelerated aging process.
- **Micronutrient Testing** - Nutritional deficiencies are often at the root of many chronic diseases and symptoms such as mood disorders, depression, anxiety, sleep disturbances, fibromyalgia, fatigue,

diabetes, and heart disease. Nutritional supplements can also be used to optimize health and fitness for athletes.

- **Adrenal Stress Profile** - This test is a measure of an individual's response to stress. It is also an important tool for pointing to adrenal imbalances that may be impacting a patient's health in the forms of fatigue, mood disorders and autoimmune disease.
- **Organic Acid Testing** - Provides a view into the body's cellular metabolic processes and the efficiency of metabolic function. Organic acids are metabolic intermediates that are produced during central energy production, detoxification, neurotransmitter breakdown, or intestinal microbial activity.
- **Comprehensive Hormone Testing** - These tests evaluate the balance of various critical hormone levels in the body to help develop an appropriate treatment plan through food supplements, bio-identical hormone therapy, and lifestyle recommendations.

- **Advanced Cardiometabolic Testing** - Traditional cholesterol testing is not adequate to assess an individual's true risk factor for heart disease. Advanced cardiometabolic testing can reveal these risk factors and direct preventive care.
- **Heavy Metal/Essential Element Testing** - We live in a very toxic world where we encounter chemical and toxins on a daily basis. Evidence suggests that chronic toxic element exposure can adversely affect: energy levels, reproductive function, cancer risk of all kinds, neurological development and function, respiratory, cardiac, liver, and immune functions, cognitive and emotional health and degenerative conditions.
- **Food Sensitivity Testing** - This test measures levels of IgG antibodies specific to anywhere from **30-200** foods causing patient reactions. IgG antibodies are associated with "non-allergic" or "delayed" food reactions that can worsen or contribute to many health conditions. The aim is to pinpoint food allergies and sensitivities that may be disrupting digestion and opening the door to autoimmune

disorders and other inflammatory diseases. It may also indicate the presence of leaky gut syndrome and other digestive issues.

- **Fasting Insulin** - Excessive Insulin in the blood is an indicator of Insulin Resistance which means cells in your muscles, fat, and liver don't respond well to insulin and cannot easily take up glucose from your blood. Long before a person is diagnosed with Type 2 Diabetes, insulin levels keep rising until the Pancreas gives up. Excessive insulin can lead to chronic disease, shortening of telomeres and advanced aging. Insulin resistance is now considered a more effective indicator of cardiovascular disease.
- **Homocysteine** - Homocysteine is a protein component and its deficiency can be linked to the decline in brain function, cardiac health and cognitive ability when coupled with a vitamin B deficiency. However higher levels are linked to detoxification defects – inability of your body to eliminate toxins - which can increase your risk for chronic diseases.

- **Inflammatory Markers** - Inflammation within the body can be determined through a blood test. This test measures biomarkers called c-reactive protein, white blood cells, and many other biochemicals, which are often linked to inflammation.
- **Oxidative Stress Markers** - These tests indicate damage to your DNA.
- **Vitamin D:** Those with a vitamin D deficiency can experience chronic illness. Alternatively, having an excess of vitamin D can also be damaging to your overall health.

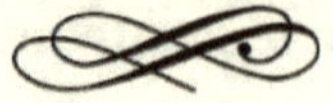

# 10. Receive Personalized Care

Based on the extensive history provided by you and the results from the functional laboratories, we will provide you a personalized plan based on the five pillars of health to ensure the systems in the body are functioning in harmony.

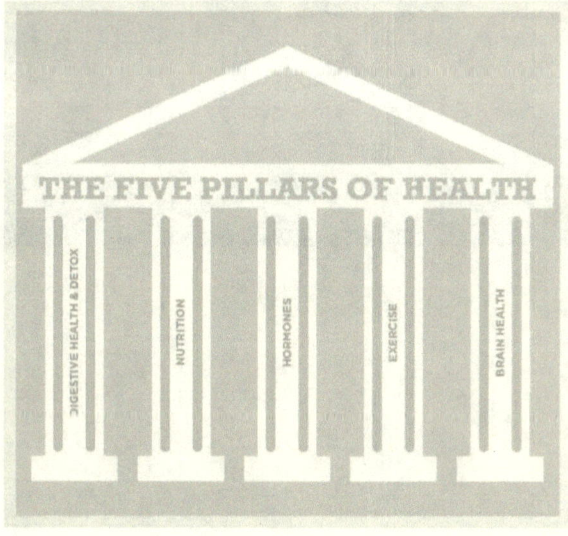

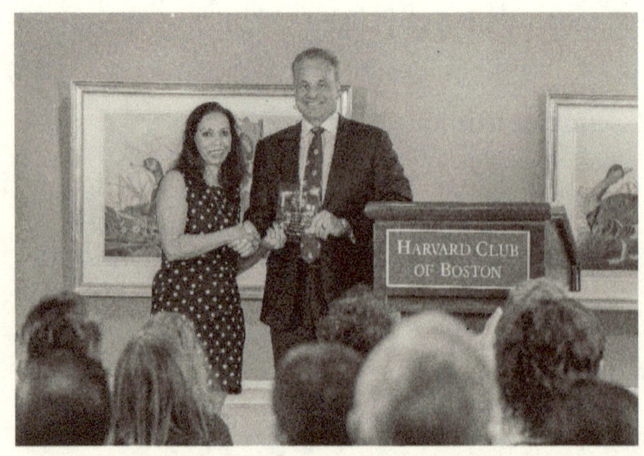
HARVARD CLUB
OF BOSTON

# Part III - The Pillars

*"Health is like money, we never have a true idea of its value until we lose it."*

# PILLAR #1 – DIGESTIVE HEALTH & DETOXIFICATION

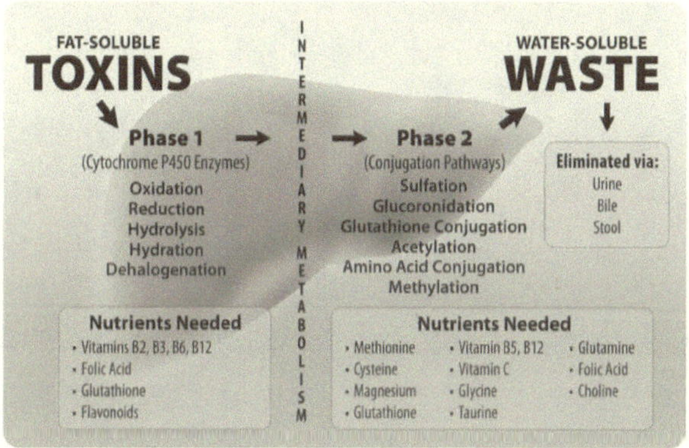


There are many fad detox diets on the market these days. Though it is important to ensure your body is getting rid of toxins, these fad diets can be very harmful to your system. It is much more beneficial to undergo a structured, medically-supervised detoxification program to greatly improve your chances of reducing ill-effects of chronic disease. The detox plan provided at Anchor Wellness Center works to remove toxins and pathogens at a cellular level with gentle support to your liver with necessary supplements.

We will also help you focus on eliminating improper food choices, pathogens and other toxins to help you start feeling better.

# PILLAR #2 - NUTRITION

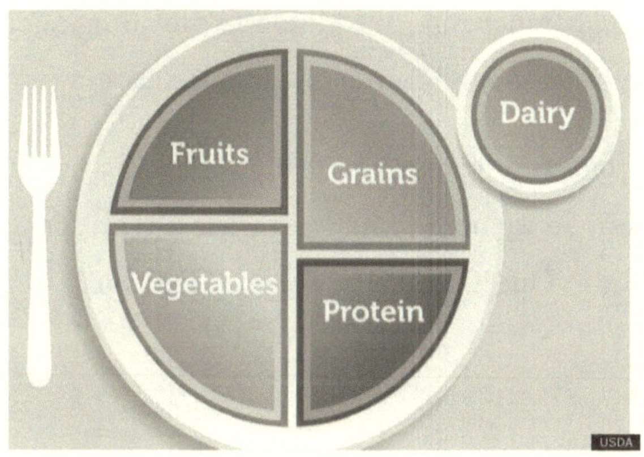


Most of us seem to live and die by the FDA approved Food pyramid, and somewhere along the way, we start looking like one. We have all heard that "You are what you eat". But I'd like to say that "You are not just what you eat but what you digest". Broccoli is generally a very healthy vegetable, but I had a patient for whom Broccoli was causing internal inflammation. It was hard for her to accept that a healthy vegetable like Broccoli – and she ate it frequently – was causing issues with her digestion. She became an instant believer when she stopped it for only a week and her symptoms disappeared.

We are learning from research in the field of *nutrigenomics*, that food components, in addition to providing calories for energy, can also modulate gene expression.

What you eat programs your body with messages of health or illness. So we need to find out what is right for you and your body. This is Nutrition designed for You!

# PILLAR #3 – HORMONAL BALANCE

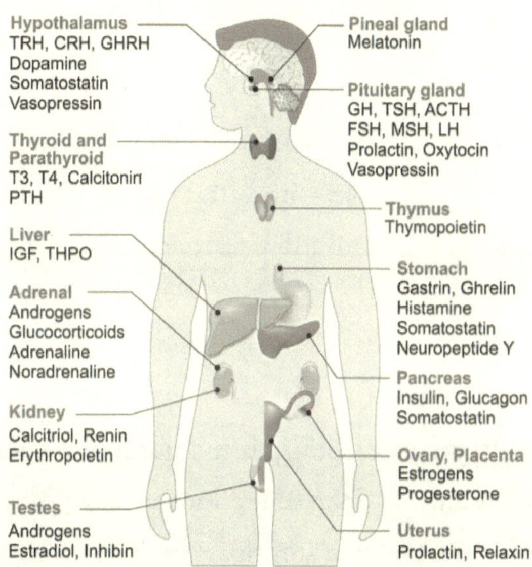


Hormones like cortisol, leptin, insulin and others affect our physical and mental health in many ways. Obesity is not necessarily due to gluttony or sloth, but it is equally likely to be a hormonal problem or a biochemical problem.

Balancing hormones is a complex process and has to done on an individual basis. Unlike traditional cookie cutter approach, Functional Medicine emphasizes a custom approach for each individual patient. Following is a summary of some of the major hormones that come into play:

**Cortisol**

This is the Master Stress hormone and is produced by our adrenal glands. It works with certain parts of our brain to control our mood, motivation, fear, fight or flight response, etc.

**Leptin**

Our fat cells produce leptin, which informs our brain to use fat stores as energy. Sometimes, human body can develop leptin resistance and start storing excess fat rather than using it as fuel to produce energy.

**Insulin**

Insulin is a critical hormone that regulates the amount of glucose in our blood stream. Sometimes human body develops insulin resistance which, if left unchecked, will eventually lead to Type II Diabetes. Studies have shown that insulin resistance maybe a prime marker for cardiovascular diseases.

With Functional Medicine, we identify the causes for insulin resistance and address them and help your body to use insulin in the proper way to help you start feeling better.

## Thyroid Dysfunction

Your thyroid glands help your body to control weight, and feel energetic among other benefits. A malfunctioning thyroid is often the main underlying culprit in Chronic diseases or dysfunction.

## Estrogen/Progesterone & Testosterone

For women it is critical to ensure there is a healthy balance of estrogen, progesterone and testosterone. We will help track your hormones for a period of time, to see any impact they are having on your overall health including weight control.

*Every time you eat or drink, you are either feeding disease or fighting it.*

# Pillar #4 - Exercise

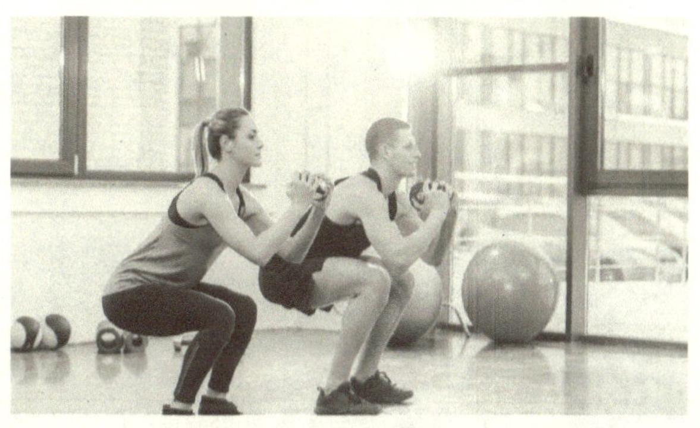

Including exercise into your daily routine is important for your body to look and feel its best. To get the best bang for your buck, you should know what exercise is the right one for your body. At Anchor Wellness Center, we will help you determine which exercise is best for you, with emphasis on High Intensity Interval Training (HIIT) to help improve overall health.

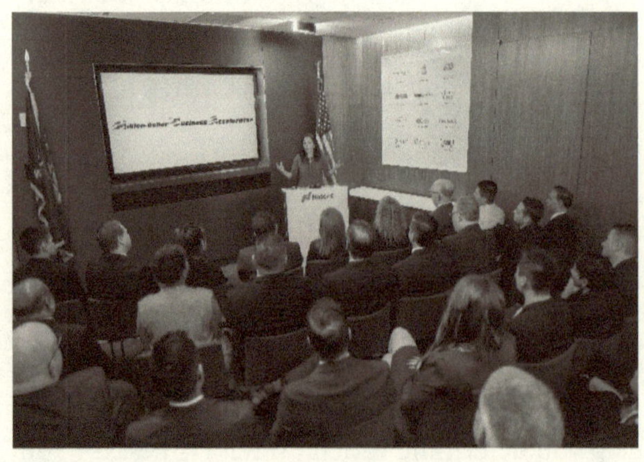

# PILLAR #5 - BRAIN HEALTH

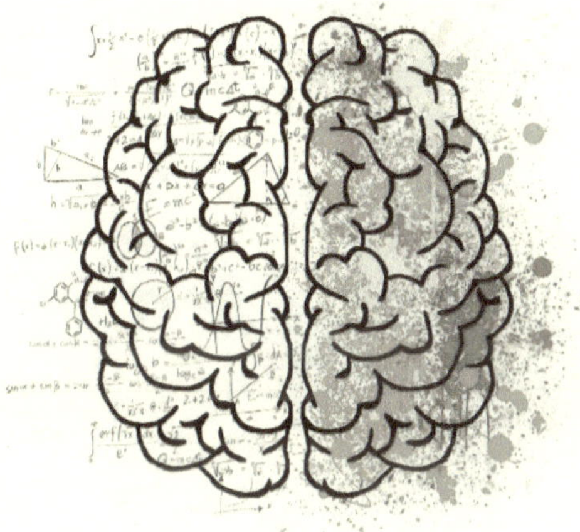

You are your brain! Your brain determines your identity and every aspect of your life and without brain, there is no self and no awareness of the world. Brain is a highly complex organ with billions of interconnected neurons to process "electrical" signals which form the basis of all skills, memories, thoughts and feelings, and most importantly - a sense of self.

We are also prone to Neurodegenerative diseases which unfortunately, have no cure. It takes years and in many cases decades for symptoms of Cognitive Decline to appear. This means your lifestyle, environment, diet, injuries, exposures, infections and more have led to this point. The only way to slow-down and potentially reverse the decline is to fix what caused it in the first place.

# THE NEXT STEP

As mentioned in the introduction, this is a summary of general guidelines towards a pathway to true health and wellness. To get a Holistic view of everything that is happening in your body and to address the root cause of any dysfunction, a comprehensive health program tailored for you and your unique chemical, hormonal, and physiological needs will be necessary for sustainable results.

If you are interested in learning more about the potential benefits of Functional Medicine for you , I invite you to schedule a complimentary 15-minute phone consultation with one of our health coaches, by calling 832-246-8437 or by emailing

info@anchorwellnesscenter.com

**A few caveats:**

First, I do not accept every request for my health program. It is essential that my clients understand that it is a therapeutic relationship between my team and them and they have to be ready to make the necessary lifestyle changes to achieve the significant impact towards their health.

*Trust me, if you are not healthy, nothing else matters.*

Second, you should know what to expect from me.

At our initial meeting, face to face or virtual, I will review your personal and family health history, your goals and expectations, perform necessary physical examinations, and look at any and all comprehensive lab tests designed to look at the body's complex systems and their functions. At the end of this meeting, I will also determine if you are a candidate for ongoing consultations. If you are a candidate and wish to proceed, I will create a customized three-to-twelve month program for your specific case and we can get started right away.

I take on a limited number of clients each month and only accept people into our program who we know we can help, and who are willing to make health their priority. We devote our time to giving personalized, one-on-one clinical care and health coaching. Our programs are tailored to the client's unique needs and goals.

It's time to stop spending on sickness and *invest in Wellness.*

So, what are you waiting for? Anchor your health in the Sea of Wellness.

Contact us today at (832) 246-8437 or email info@anchorwellnesscenter.com with any questions and to claim your spot for a personalized health evaluation.

Sincerely,

Minni Malhotra, M.D., ABFM, ABAARM, IFMCP

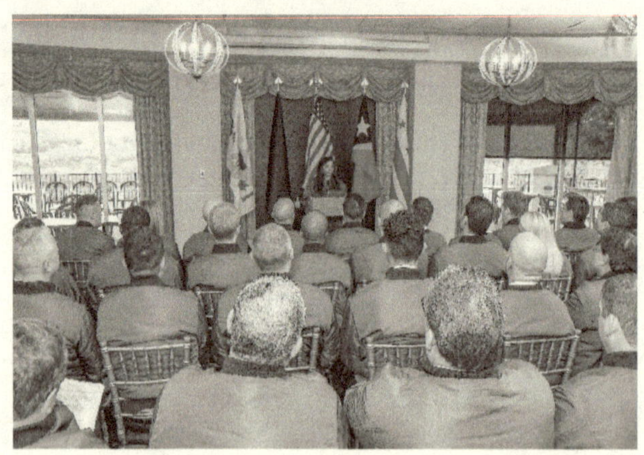

# FAQS

**Why do I need a wellness a program?**

Generally speaking, chronic ailments are caused by a systematic failure and long-term disturbances in the human body. It takes time and detailed-testing to identify the triggers and tease out the factors that keep you sick: toxins, hormonal imbalance, inflammation, digestive dysfunction, and psychological considerations. You become a partner with us and our team supports you to help attain the mutually determined goal.

**What should I expect during this partnership?**

Your journey to health will be designed based on your unique situation. We start off by sending you via e-mail a detailed history form called the Living Matrix. This needs to be filled prior to your initial visit to help identify the starting point of your healing process.

**Do you accept insurance for office visits?**

We do not accept insurance for office visits. Upon request, we can provide you with a copy of your invoices which YOU can submit to your insurance company. We cannot guarantee what reimbursement, if any, you may receive. We do not submit claims or directly call insurance companies on your behalf.

**Do you accept insurance for testing?**

Sometimes. In most cases, for standard lab testing, your insurance can be billed directly by the labs. Some specialty labs may not be covered by your insurance plans. Please check with your insurance company regarding deductibles and reimbursement for out-of-network labs.

**What testing do you use?**

We are constantly updating the functional medicine tests we offer based on emerging scientific data.

**What tests will I get?**

Every plan is unique. We work with you to customize testing orders based on your health needs and personal preferences.

**Do you accept Medicare?**

We do not participate with Medicare, nor do we bill Medicare.

**What form of payments are accepted?**

You may pay by check, credit card, or HSA debit card.

**Do you offer payment plans?**

We do offer payment plans for our programs depending on patients' needs and circumstances.

**Will Dr. Minni be my primary care physician?**

Dr. Minni Malhotra is board certified in Family Medicine and she will be able to address all of your health care needs. However, she cannot function as your primary care provider (PCP) for insurance purposes. If you do not have a PCP, she will recommend one for you. She has worked with many of the excellent doctors who understand what she does and are willing to support you in your healing care.

**Can I consult with Dr. Minni if I live outside of The Woodlands, TX?**

Yes of course! Consults can be done virtually from anywhere through our HIPPA compliant platform. We have patients all over the country and even overseas.

**What does being board certified in Anti-Aging and Regenerative Medicine mean?**

**Please visit**

**www.a4m.com**

**What is Functional Medicine?**

Functional Medicine's primary focus is on finding root cause and treatment of various chronic ailments by taking an integrative approach encompassing environmental, mind-body connections and genetic considerations. To learn more

https://www.functionalmedicine.org/What_is_Functional_Medicine/AboutFM/

**Is Dr. Minni available for speaking events?**

Yes of course. Dr. Minni has been participating in educational and speaking engagements for quite some time. She has shared her message through a TEDx talk which is available worldwide on Youtube thru TEDx platform. She has also shared her message at Harvard Club of Boston, has been on stage with Suzzane Sommers and many others. It is her passion to educate the community and create an awareness of true healing, and the empowerment each person has to remain healthy.

**What is the price of a Program or Membership?**

Prices are quoted individually as functional medicine is never a one-size-fits-all approach. You will receive a program price at the end of your new patient wellness consultation based on your health goals and needs.

**Can I bring a friend or family member to the appointment?**

Absolutely. However, we ask you to find childcare for any small children or infants as the appointments are lengthy.

**How many visits will I need?**

This depends on the complexity of your problem. We typically require a 3 to 6 month engagement to affect a meaningful change in your health and overall sense of well-being.

## How do I schedule an appointment?

Please call our office directly to schedule your new patient wellness consultation.

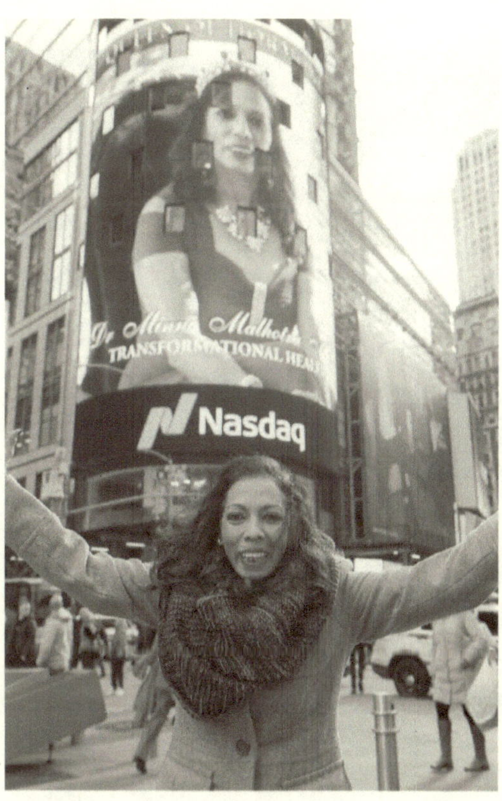

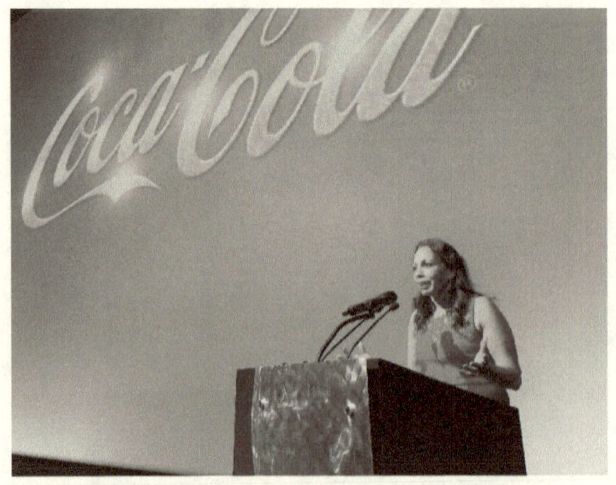
Coca-Cola

# ABOUT THE AUTHOR

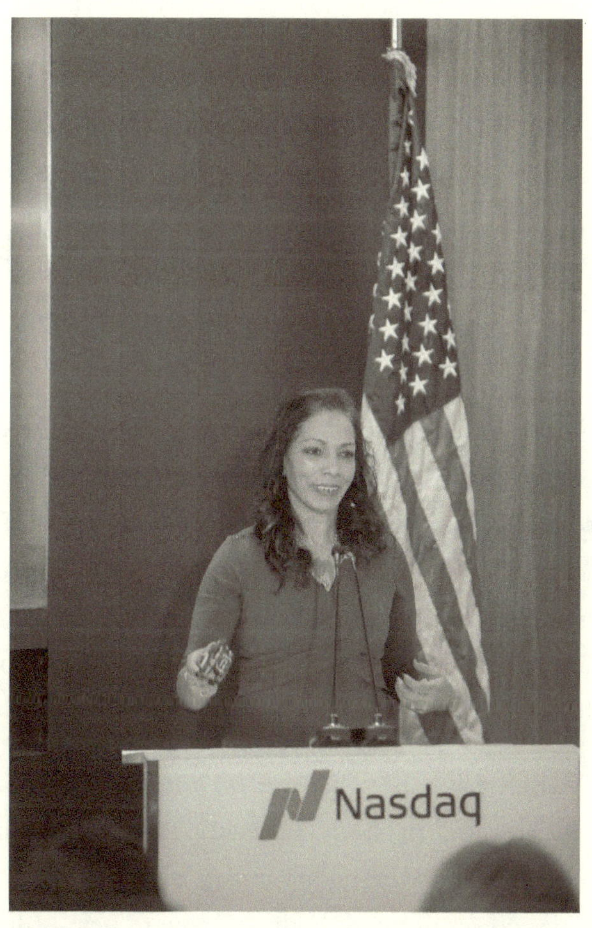

Dr. Minni Malhotra is a Wife, a Mother, Author but her most coveted accomplishment is being a Healer. Her passion for helping people led her to become a Physician. During her traditional medicine practice for more than 20 years(10 years in the USA in addition to a previous 10 years in India) she realized she was not really curing her patients but just putting band aids. Recognizing that healthcare in our country has turned into a disease-care system rather than healthcare management, she has actively trained to help people attain lifelong health and wellness through natural treatment.

In addition to Board certification from American Academy of Family Medicine, she is also certified with American Board of Anti-Aging and Regenerative Medicine. She is also a Certified Practitioner with Institute of Functional Medicine. In her quest for knowledge to help her patients, she is currently pursuing training in Homeopathic Medicine.

Dr. Malhotra is a firm believer of Integrative medicine - appropriate use of both conventional and alternative methods facilitates the body's innate healing response and using the power of mind, body and soul to help us heal. It is an evidence-based approach which emphasizes the therapeutic relationship between practitioner and patient. She incorporates the best diagnostic tools and technologies from conventional medicine, as well as emerging tests and tools that help us identify the critical imbalances that are at the root of all illness. Rather than simply treating symptoms and/or merely managing a health condition by camouflaging symptoms with medications, she aims to resolve the root cause of the problem. She believes in patient-centered and not disease-centered, medicine.

# Notes

# NOTES

# Notes

# Notes

# Notes

# Notes

# Notes

# NOTES

# Notes

# Notes

www.ingramcontent.com/pod-product-compliance
Lightning Source LLC
LaVergne TN
LVHW050936080826
845145LV00004B/1285

* 9 7 8 0 9 9 6 3 1 9 7 9 9 *